Mediterranean Diet Cookbook

The Essential beginners guide for Men and Women to Weight loss and Lower Your Blood Pressure and Improve Your Health

(Delicious Recipes for the Ultimate Healthy Lifestyle)

Karen Moran

Published by Jason Thawne Publishing House

© Karen Moran

Mediterranean Diet Cookbook: The Essential beginners guide for Men and Women to Weight loss and Lower Your Blood Pressure and Improve Your Health (Delicious Recipes for the Ultimate Healthy Lifestyle)

All Rights Reserved

ISBN 978-1-989749-84-5

This document is geared towards providing exact and reliable information in regards to the topic and issue covered. The publication is sold with the idea that the publisher isn't required to render accounting, officially permitted, or otherwise, qualified services. If advice is necessary, legal or even professional, a practiced individual in the profession should be ordered.

- From a Declaration of Principles which was accepted and approved equally by a Committee of the American Bar Association and a Committee of Publishers and Associations.

In no way is it legal to reproduce, duplicate, or even transmit any part of this document in either electronic means or in printed format. Recording of this publication is strictly prohibited and any storage of this document isn't allowed unless with proper written permission from the publisher. All rights reserved.

The information provided herein is stated to be truthful and consistent, in that any liability, in terms of inattention or otherwise, by any usage or abuse of any policies, processes, or directions contained within is the solitary and also utter responsibility of the recipient reader. Under no circumstances will any legal responsibility or blame be held against the publisher for any reparation, damages, or monetary loss due to the information herein, either directly or indirectly.

Respective authors own all copyrights not held by the publisher.

The information herein is offered for just informational purposes solely, and is universal as so. The presentation of the information is without contract or any type of guarantee assurance.

The trademarks that are used are without any consent, and also the publication of the trademark is without permission or backing by the trademark owner. All trademarks and brands within this book are for clarifying purposes only and are the owned by the owners themselves, not affiliated with this document.

TABLE OF CONTENTS

Part 1 1

Introduction 2

Chapter 1: Eating The Mediterranean Way 4

Chapter 2: A Successful Plan For You 11

Chapter 3: Adapting The Perfect Diet Plan 17

Chapter 4: Beautiful Breakfast Recipes 21

Sparta Oatmeal 21

Chickpea Hash Browns 22

Greek Honey Yogurt With Dates 23

Whole Grain Healthy Pancakes 24

Greek Yoghurt And Berry Surprise 25

Oatmeal With Banana And Nut Topping 26

Toastie With Avocado 27

Cinnamon And Fruity Couscous 27

Flavorsome Feta Frittata 28

Chapter 5: Sumptuous Snacks 31

Dip In A Glass 31

Crunchy Crackers With Feta 32

Berry And Ricotta Tasty 33

Spiced Veggie Hummus Dips 33

Tasty Salad 34

Tuna Pockets 35

Chickpeas And Couscous.. 36

Chapter 6: Magnificent Mains..................................... 38

Cauliflower Italian Style 39

Oven Roasted Chicken Le Mediterranean................. 40

South Med Shrimp... 41

Brown Rice With Feta Cheese 42

Minestrone Stew 43

Mediterranean Meatballs 45

Greek Chicken... 46

Spicy Mediterranean Fillets... 47

Mediterranean Spaghetti... 48

Steamed Mussels... 49

Chapter 7: Daring Desserts... 51

Sushi Dessert 51

Pudding-Rice With Fruit 52

Panna Delight 54

Italian Stuffed Apples... 55

Nut Peach Boats 55

Lemon Pudding.. 56

Baklava With Cinnamon.. 58

Tiramisu 59

Luscious Berries And Greek Yogurt 61

Chapter 8: Long Term Weight Loss And Heart Smart Achievability 62

Conclusion 68

Part 2 70

Introduction 71

Stuffed Tomatoes 76

Greek-Style Picnic Salad 79

Chicken-Garbanzo Salad 82

Mediterranean Egg Scramble 84

Zucchini And Goat Cheese Frittata 87

Coconut Cookies 89

Peach Melba 90

Apple Strudel 91

Cherry Clafoutis 93

Apricot Rosemary Muffins 94

Minty Fruit Salad 96

Upside Down Apricot Cake 97

Greek Yogurt Pie 98

Butternut Squash Crumble 100

Healthy Chocolate Mousse 101

- Red Wine Poached Pears 103
- Baked Peaches With Amaretti 104
- Orange Spiced Apricot Compote 105
- Coffee Granita 107
- Sweet Couscous Salad 108
- Orange Olive Oil Cake 110
- Spiced Walnut Cake 111
- Raisins Honey Baked Donuts 113
- Roasted Figs With Rosemary And Yogurt 115
- Ham Spinach Pork Roulade 116
- Salmon With Salsa Verde 119
- Baked Sea Bass With Potatoes And Coriander 120
- Cherry Tomato Caper Chicken 122
- Eggplant Ragout Spaghetti 123
- Mediterranean Diet 126
- Conclusion 127
- About The Author 127

Part 1

Introduction

Back in the 1960s, people in the Mediterranean were observed to be living a lot healthier than Americans and other natives from other countries of the same age. They were also less susceptible to many killer diseases and illnesses. Since the 1960s and to the current times, many studies have been carried out. The research definitively shows, that the Mediterranean diet can: help with weight loss, aid in the prevention of heart attacks, strokes and type 2 diabetes. All of which can all lead to premature death and or decreased quality of life.

The diet is a heart-healthy eating plan which aims to fulfill your appetite, rather than make you feel deprived after or between meal times. Most healthy diets are based on whole grains, fruit, vegetables, and fish. After careful analysis, it has been shown, with minor variations in the quantities of the proportions of some foods - the risk of heart disease can be reduced, massively.

A lot of diets aim to reduce fats and oils in the diet, but the Mediterranean diet actually encourages both (in small amounts). So, to follow the characteristics of Mediterranean cooking, and also have the ability to have meals with friends is a bonus! Many of them may not even realize you are on a diet. Throughout the book, I will give you all that you need to know about feeling healthy and revived through correct eating, the Mediterranean way...

Chapter 1: Eating the Mediterranean Way

The Mediterranean is a large area consisting of many different countries, so not all the same foods are eaten by the same nationalities, which shows us that the benefits are not only coming from certain foods in this diet. Actually, the benefits are coming from eating a certain way and the foods together. This can vastly increase what types of foods you can eat, and not leave you with a limited grocery list, during the process.

I will explain in more detail what the Mediterranean diet consists of and the what you can eat (including the things that you must limit or avoid altogether). So please remember that all the information given is only a guideline, and the plans and recipes given can be adjusted for your personal preferences. As with all diets, if you have any doubts or are on any medication, always consult your doctor before commencement.

Regular Eating

Vegetables: Cucumber, Carrots, Cauliflower, Tomatoes, Broccoli, Kale, Onions and Spinach plus others.

Seeds and Nuts: Almonds, Walnuts, Sunflower, Pumpkin and Cashews etc.

Tubers: Potatoes, Turnips and Sweet Potatoes etc.

Poultry: Chicken, Turkey or Duck.

Whole Grains: Whole Grain Bread, Pasta, Barley, Corn and Brown Rice plus others.

Note: in the Mediterranean, bread is normally only used for dipping and not used in sandwiches.

Herbs and Spices: Garlic, Rosemary, Sage, Pepper etc.

Fish and Seafood: Mackerel, Trout, Salmon, Shrimp, Prawns, Mussels etc.

Fruits: Apples, Oranges, Pears, Figs, Dates, Avocados and any Berries plus many more.

Legumes: Beans, Peas, Lentils and Chickpeas etc.

Good Fats and Oils: Extra Virgin Olive Oil and Olives, Avocado Oil.

Moderate Eating

Yogurt, cheese, poultry and eggs.

Less frequent eating and red meats.

Things to Avoid

Processed foods – Low fat, diet or ready meals.

Processed meats – Hot dogs or sausages etc.

Trans fats – These are found in processed foods and margarine.

Refined grains – Anything made with refined wheat, white bread, pasta etc.

Refined oils – Canola oil, soybean oil etc.

Sugary things – Sugar for tea, coffee, sodas, candy, ice cream.

Drinks

Compared to most diets, coffee and tea are accepted and the recommended amount of red wine per day is one glass. Water should be consumed throughout the day to keep you hydrated, plus it helps to flush out your system. Fruit Juices and sweetened drinks should be avoided as they contain extra sugar.

Snacks

With the Mediterranean way of eating you normally only eat three times per day, although if you get hungry between meals here are a few things that you can have as a snack: half a cup of nuts, half a cup of berries, raw carrots, and fruit.

Dining Out on the Mediterranean Diet

If dining out at restaurants, you will probably realize this is one of the easiest diets cater for, so here are a few tips on how to make your meal suitable.

Order whole grain bread and instead of butter ask if they have olive oil for spreading. Ask if they can fry your food in olive oil, or if there is the possibility of having the food steamed. Choose fish or seafood for your main course.

The general principles are not to give a quick fix or to starve your body of certain foods that are required for normal day to day activity. The purpose is to give healthy eating on a daily basis - this of which has no adverse effects if followed over the long term like some diets.

As a general rule, you should aim to maximize your intake of any of the foods that are in the eat frequently section e.g. fruits, vegetables, legumes and wholegrain cereals. Limit the amount of salt used for flavoring when cooking, because the increased amount has been directly linked to high blood pressure. The alternatives to flavoring by using salt are herbs and spices, and also garlic.

The countries in the Mediterranean include Greece, Spain and southern Italy being the main ones. After you have seen and tried some of the recipes in this book, it is simple to find more healthy variations from these countries. So, you will soon realize with a slight adaption they can fit into your diet with ease as most recipes are already diet friendly. You will also notice the recipes contain high amounts of legume consumption, this is recommended on a regular level along with unrefined cereals, fruits and vegetables, especially leafy green vegetables, too. And all of them have increased amounts of olive oil, either for cooking or to add flavor to your dishes.

You will also notice, most recipes call for fish or seafood, and this is recommended above poultry and red meats. Many studies have shown the main contributing factor to the benefits of the diet is actually the olive oil, of which you should aim to use Extra Virgin Olive Oil, where possible. And although slightly more expensive, it is a much higher quality - as it is the purest oil that comes from the first pressing of the olives. It is said that olive oil may lower the risks of all mortality cancers, cardiovascular disease and other chronic diseases, as well.

Although there are many countries around the Mediterranean, this diet takes a broad overview of foods and recipes available from all these countries plus others. I have tried to not limit the recipes to one particular country. You will also notice you can have 2 small glasses of red wine or 1 large glass per day, and studies show that this can also help decrease the risk of heart disease, stroke, diabetes and early death.

Please note, drinking more than this amount can actually increase the risks of the illnesses that a small amount helps to cure. Although this diet has been around for many years, there is the Mediterranean Diet Foundation which is based in Barcelona, where they still continue to study the benefits of the Mediterranean diet. It is also important to note that their aim is to promote investigation of health, historical, cultural and gastronomic aspects of the Mediterranean Diet. As with their own studies, they also analyze the scientific results of tests that others have conducted, in accordance to regulatory guidelines. It shows how important the people of the Mediterranean take this diet, as this foundation was first established in 1996.

If you are interested, you can search for more exclusive information regarding this amazing diet online. Sometimes you need to see the results or stories of others to believe that they are true. In saying that, there are also well backed research results which can be looked at in conjunction with this information. I want you to have the entire picture, so you can see for yourself.

Chapter 2: A Successful Plan for You

With most diets, you are encouraged to do regular exercise which helps to burn calories. Not only is this tiring and time consuming but it is also slightly misleading, because the benefits you are getting are from the diet and not just from extra exercise you are doing. As the Mediterranean diet is a well-balanced diet without many food items having to be omitted, you do not have to do much additional exercise to what you would normally do, although it is recommended to have an exercise regime in place or to keep physically active, for health promotion.

Although after a while you will be doing this anyway, as you will feel more energetic naturally. As the majority of the food items on the Mediterranean diet are fruits and vegetables (with limited amounts of red meats and dairy and poultry), most of these are absorbed and digested by the body a lot quicker, so not only are the nutrients absorbed faster, but there will be nothing making you feel overly bloated after meal times.

The best way to plan your diet is on a weekly basis, this way you can easily monitor your intake of dairy and red meats, these you can save for dining out with friends to make you evening more enjoyable. When planning your meals, you should choose a varied menu and try to include fish and seafood two to three times per week if not more. Iron would be substituted via vitamins, if you are anemic.

To keep physically active, it is recommended you either start a new sport or go dancing, there is no need for strenuous trips to the gym. To make this easier it is best to enlist the help of a partner or a friend, as this will take away the thought of starting something new with a lot of strangers.

A few sample exercises you can do at home are:

Bodyweight Squats

Stand as straight as you can with feet apart slightly wider than shoulder width.

Hold arms straight in front of you at shoulder level.

Brace your abs and lower your body as far as you can by bending your knees.

Repeat a few times until you can do it more easily and then do about 20 repetitions.

Hip Raise

Lay flat on the floor with your knees bent and your feet are flat, and place your arms at a 45-degree angle with palms facing up.

Hold your stomach in and hold it in, this gives you a tight core, and breathe normally and then raise your hips so your body forms a straight line when raised. Pause for 5 seconds then lower back to the starting position. Once you have got used to this, do 10 repetitions at a time.

These are just a couple of easy exercises you can do a couple of times per day as they don't take too much time to do, maybe 15 minutes in a morning and 15 minutes in an evening. This would be the full allocation of exercise that is recommended on a daily basis, and that is without too much exertion or without any other activities you do.

Time Management

As we have mentioned, the Mediterranean diet will lead to a change in eating habits and lifestyle and is generally based on 3 good meals a day. For this reason, you should aim to give yourself time to actually fit these meal times into your day. If you are extra busy and only have time for a snack, you will feel deprived after eating. So you will become hungry before your next meal and will have the urge to snack, not only this, you will have missed out on the nutrients that one of the lunch dishes would have given you.

When doing your weekly plan, if you can allocate the times for your morning exercise, breakfast, lunch, dinner and evening activities and stick to this, the whole routine will become a habit. Not only will you feel better and less hungry, but you will start to do these things without having to think about it - so you will have less urge to snack in between meals. The other benefit of sticking to your routine is, if you happen to slip on your meals or routine, it will not have as much effect, if it occurs sometimes. Always try to keep your routine, though.

Staying Focused

In the start as with most diets, you can be tempted to slip - which would lead to quitting all your hard work. When and if you find yourself hungry between meals it is recommended to have a piece of fruit or a small handful of nuts - as these are on your, "eat regularly" list of foods. Other tips are to drink lots of water throughout the day, as this will keep you hydrated and also stave off hunger.

If you are on the Mediterranean diet with the aim to lose weight, try not to weigh yourself daily and only do it once per week if you must. Your body can fluctuate throughout the day, especially if you have been drinking lots of water, and this would still be in your system and show up when you are on the scales. Aim to get a good night's sleep, and remember that sitting on the couch and watching too much TV gives unnecessary distractions. This may lead into the temptation to snack, even if you are not really hungry. Chewing sugarless chewing gum is also another tip to stop you feeling hungry, as this will keep your mind and mouth occupied. One final tip is to keep a diary of everything that you eat and drink, this will make you aware of how much you are physically consuming. Also, studies have shown people who keep a diary tend to lose more weight than people who don't.

As a final comment, you should try to enjoy your diet and don't think of it as a chore that has to be done, if it is enjoyable it will become easier. So make it fun, and have fun while you do it. It can be a total lifestyle change, which is recommended for longevity in health, and for your heart, as well.

Chapter 3: Adapting the Perfect Diet Plan
As the Mediterranean diet is primarily a vegetable and fruit diet it is quite easy to adapt to, for meals not containing meat. Meals containing meat can be altered to use legumes, and more nuts and seeds and soy based products. The diet pyramid also puts emphasis on whole grains as part of the daily diet with fats playing a small part. If you adapt the diet for no meat, it is advisable to increase your intake of unsalted nuts to one handful per day - to counteract the loss of protein you would be getting from fish and poultry etc. You could also use dried beans, tempeh or tofu based products and also non-fat dairy products. It is also recommended to eat your maximum allocation of eggs and cheese on a daily or weekly basis.

Some considerations must be noted, if your diet consists of no meat or fish, it is also advisable to take fish oil supplements to boost your intake of omega-3 fatty acids which are found in seafood, because this also helps maintain the cardiovascular benefits you will gain from being on the

Mediterranean diet. As you will lose some vitamin D, it is advisable to make sure all the dairy products you consume are fortified with Vitamin D, and also combine your bean dishes with generous servings of leafy green vegetables and tomatoes. The extra vitamin C you will gain from the vegetables helps to absorb the iron that is provided by the beans. Spending more time in sunlight will also increase your intake of vitamin D. As a general rule, vegetarians that are on the Mediterranean diet should aim to have at least six portions of fruit and vegetables per day, with whole grain cereals, bread and pasta eaten at every meal.

As it is advised throughout the diet, you should omit the use of butter and instead replace it with olive oil when cooking - or use it to flavor bread and also as a combination which can be used as a dip.

If you are vegetarian it is advisable to pay a visit to your doctor before commencing, so they can advise what you can do to boost your intake of vitamin B-12.

If you are vegan and also wish to try the Mediterranean diet, this is also possible and easy to adapt the recipes to include no animal products. Some recommendations are as follows:

Have larger servings of whole grains and vegetables, beans are of a significant importance as they lower blood cholesterol levels and are linked to improved blood glucose. Add a little extra virgin olive oil onto your vegetables which can help with the absorption of some compounds.

Flavor your dishes by using nuts and seeds, as this also adds texture so your mouthfuls are more interesting. Herbs and spices can improve flavor and also provide protective phytonutrients.

For your food supplements consider DHA and EPA, these are long chain Omega-3 fatty acids which are found in fatty fish. These can also be purchased in non-gel capsules with the nutrients coming from algae-based products - which contain no traces of animal products. As with the vegetarians, it is advisable to keep active, enjoy the sunlight and make the most of your healthy lifestyle.

If you like meat in your diet it is advisable to follow what is laid out in the food pyramid and limit your red meat intake. Then when you do this, your portion of meat should only be the size of a pack of playing cards. It is also recommended not to eat fatty meats like sausages and bacon, as this type of fat are non-healthy fats and have no benefit to your system (and just lay in your stomach).

It is highly recommended you swap some of your red meat meals for poultry dishes, although these are recommended to be limited, so the best solution is to increase the amount of seafood and fish you consume, and save your red meat or poultry dish for special occasions. Or incorporate them only twice or three times per week, essentially.

Chapter 4: Beautiful Breakfast Recipes

Sparta Oatmeal

Serves 1
Ingredients
¼ cup cut oats
1 sprig parsley (chopped)
4 dates (chopped)
3 tbsp. olive oil
Salt and pepper (to taste)
¼ cup shallots (chopped)
2 slices tofu, 2 cups dates
Bacon 2 slices
Instructions
Cook the oats by instructions on the packet, sauté the shallots, bacon, and shallots, until soft, add rosemary and stir until all mixture is combined add salt and pepper to taste.
Transfer to dish.
Serve warm.

Chickpea Hash Browns

Serves 2

Ingredients

2 cups frozen hash browns
¼ cup chopped onion
¼ tsp salt
2 large eggs organic or free range
½ tbsp. ginger minced or grated
1/8 cup extra virgin olive oil
7 ½ oz. (½ can) chickpeas
½ cup zucchini chopped
1 tsp chili (can also use curry powder ½ tbsp.)
1 cup finely chopped leafy greens (kale, baby spinach or cabbage can be used)

Instructions

In a large bowl combine the hash browns, leafy greens, ginger, chili powder, and salt.
Heat oil in a skillet over medium heat.
Add mixture and press until level and flat.
Cook until golden brown on the bottom.
Reduce heat to low temperature.
Break the potato mixture then add the zucchini and chickpeas until combined.
Press flat again and make 4 indentations in the mixture.

Crack eggs and pour 1 into each dent, cover and cook until eggs are set. This should be 4 – 5 minutes for runny yolks.

Greek Honey Yogurt with Dates

Serves 1
Ingredients
1 small carton Greek yogurt
¼ cup pitted dates chopped
1 tbsp. honey
Instructions
Place yogurt in small dish.
Pour on chopped dates and combine.
Drizzle with honey.

Whole Grain Healthy Pancakes

Makes 2 large pancakes – double quantities to make more

Ingredients

½ cup oats

½ tsp baking soda

1/8 tsp salt

1 tbsp. canola oil

1 tbsp. honey (agave can be used)

1 cup Greek-style yogurt (either plain or vanilla)

1 large egg

¼ cup all-purpose flour

1 tbsp. flax seeds

Optional for Toppings

Fruit or syrup or any other from your allowed foods.

Instructions

In a blender pulse the oats, flour, flax seeds, baking soda and salt for about 30 seconds.

Add the yogurt and egg, oil and honey then blend until you have a smooth batter.

Let batter stand for about 20 minutes or until thickened.

Heat a non-stick skillet over medium heat and coat surface thinly with oil.

Pour half the mixture into the skillet and cook until golden brown on the bottom and bubbles start to form on the top surface approx. 2 minutes. Flip your pancake and cook for another 2 minutes.

Cook remaining half of the batter then transfer to plates and serve warm with your toppings, re-oil pan if required.

If pancakes are too large, just reduce quantity into the skillet, approx. ¼ cup.

Greek Yoghurt and Berry Surprise
Serves 1
Ingredients
6 oz. Greek yogurt
¼ cup berries
3 tbsp. low fat granola
honey
Instructions

In a tall glass place 1/3 of the yogurt followed by 1 tbsp. granola and cover with berries.
Cover berries with yogurt and granola.
Repeat until you have used all the ingredients then drizzle with honey.

Oatmeal with Banana and Nut Topping

Ingredients
2 peeled bananas
4 tbsp. chopped walnuts or almonds any other nuts can be used
½ cup cooking oats
1 cup skimmed milk
2 tsp flax seeds
6 tbsp. honey

Instructions
Place in a microwave safe bowl the bananas and mash with a fork.
Add milk, cooking oats, flax seeds, nuts and honey, stir mixture until well combined.
Cook in microwave on high for 2 minutes.
Divide into bowls and serve hot.

Toastie with Avocado

Serves 1

Ingredients

2 large slices whole grain bread

1 small avocado

Lemon juice (to taste)

40 grams of feta cheese (crumbled)

2 thin slices ham

1 egg (organic or free range)

Fresh herbs (any of your choice)

Instructions

In a bowl place the avocado and smash with a fork, add lemon juice to taste.

Toast bread until golden then spoon mixture onto the toast, top with the cheese and ham and serve hot.

If using egg, place on top of ham and garnish with fresh herbs.

Cinnamon and Fruity Couscous

Makes 2

Ingredients

½ cup uncooked couscous (whole-wheat)

1 ½ cups low-fat milk

2 tsp olive oil
2-inch cinnamon stick (or cinnamon powder to taste)
3 tsp dark brown sugar
1/8 tsp salt
1/8 cup currants or raisins
¼ cup dried fruit chopped

Instructions

In a large saucepan heat milk and cinnamon on medium- high heat until small bubbles start to form around the edge.

Remove from heat and stir in couscous, currants, dried fruit of choice and 2 tsp of the sugar and the salt.

Cover and stand for 15 minutes.

If using cinnamon stick remove and divide into bowls, top with remaining butter and sugar, serve immediately.

Flavorsome Feta Frittata

Ingredients
½ cup crumbled feta cheese
3 tbsp. grated parmesan cheese

½ cup chopped red peppers
1 cup chopped onion
2 cloves grated or minced garlic
3 tbsp. olive oil
8 large organic or free-range eggs (beaten)
¼ cup half and half light cream and full fat milk
½ cup pitted olives
¼ cup fresh basil (chopped)
½ tsp ground black pepper
½ cup crushed onion and garlic flavored croutons

Instructions

Preheat broiler to temperature, medium high.

In broiler proof skillet heat oil and sauté onion and garlic until tender.

In large bowl beat eggs and the half and half.

Stir in peppers, olives, basil black pepper and feta cheese.

Pour mixture over the onion and garlic cook over medium heat until mixture starts to set.

Lift edge of frittata from side of skillet so wet mixture can run underneath, continue cooking until all mixture is nearly set, top most surface will still be moist, lower heat to avoid burning.

In a small bowl, crush the croutons and parmesan cheese with the remaining oil, sprinkle over the top of the frittata and broil on the top half of broiler until the top surface has set and the crouton crumbs are golden brown.

Divide between plates and serve hot.

Chapter 5: Sumptuous Snacks

Salad Skewers

Ingredients

1/3 cup olives

1/3 cup grape tomatoes small cherry tomatoes can be used

¼ seedless cucumber

Cocktail sticks

Instructions

On each cocktail stick, place 1 olive, 1 tomato and ½ slice of cucumber.

Serve with your favorite dip.

Dip in a Glass

Ingredients

3 oz. Greek yogurt plain

1 tbsp. fresh parsley chopped finely

½ cup humus

1 tsp lemon juice

2 medium tomatoes (de-seeded and chopped)

1/3 cup cucumber (de-seeded and chopped)

1/3 cup green olives (chopped)
¼ cup feta cheese (crumbled)
1 pinch salt
3 tbsp. onion (chopped)
Sliced veggies or whole meal pita bread (to be used for dipping)

Instructions

Into each serving glass layer 2 tbsp. humus, 1 tbsp. tomato, 1 tbsp. cucumber, 1 tbsp. olives and half tbsp. onion and top with 1 large tbsp. of yogurt mixture.

In a small bowl mix feta cheese, parsley, lemon juice, salt and yogurt.

Serve with vegetable strips and pita slices.

Crunchy Crackers with Feta

Ingredients

Black pepper to taste
Pinch of red pepper flakes
Garlic 2 cloves thinly sliced
Pitted olives 1 cup sliced
Feta cheese ½ cup diced
Olive oil 2 tbsp.
Lemon zest and juice of 1 lemon
Rosemary 1 tsp fresh and chopped

Instructions

In a bowl mix all the ingredients, cover and place in the refrigerator for up to one day. When ready to serve, place a small spoonful on a whole wheat cracker.

Berry and Ricotta Tasty
Ingredients
Any berries ¾ cup
Ricotta cheese 2 tbsp.
Mixed nuts 1 tbsp. (toasted and crushed)
Instructions
Place nuts in food processor and pulse until fine crumbs appear.
Place berries in a microwave bowl.
Heat berries until warm 1 to 2 minutes.
Place ricotta cheese onto the warm berries and top with the crushed nuts.

Spiced Veggie Hummus Dips
Ingredients
1 tbsp. olive oil
1 small serving humus
1 medium carrot

½ medium cucumber
½ medium red bell pepper
1 pinch paprika
1 pinch cayenne pepper

Instructions

Place hummus in small serving bowl and stir in 1 pinch of paprika and 1 pinch of cayenne pepper. Add 1 tbsp. olive oil.
Peel carrot and slice thinly.
Cut the cucumber into thin strips.
De-seed 1 red pepper and slice 1 half into thin strips.
Dip vegetables in humus and enjoy.

Tasty Salad

Serves 4

Ingredients

1 head of lettuce (any variety of choice)
2 medium tomatoes (cut into wedges)
¼ cup pitted olives sliced (any variety of olives can be used)
¼ cup crumbled feta cheese

1 medium green pepper (de-seeded and thinly sliced)
1 medium red pepper (de-seeded and thinly sliced)
Salad Dressing
1 tbsp. olive oil
3 tbsp. lemon juice
½ tsp finely chopped oregano
½ tsp finely chopped cilantro
¼ tsp black pepper
Instructions
Prepare dressing – in a small jar combine lemon juice, olive oil, oregano, cilantro, and pepper and shake well.
Wash and dry lettuce leaves and place in salad bowl.
Add bell peppers, tomatoes, olives and feta cheese then pour over the dressing.
Gently toss to coat everything.

Tuna Pockets

Ingredients

1 whole wheat pitta bread
1 tbsp. olive oil
2 lettuce leaves any variety
¼ cucumber sliced
1 medium tomato sliced
1 small onion sliced
½ can tuna chunks
Salt to taste
Pepper to taste
Instructions
In a small bowl break the tuna chunks, add olive oil.
Toast pitta bread and cut into 2.
Open pitta bread and insert lettuce, tomato, cucumber and onion along with half the tuna.
Sprinkle with salt and pepper if required.

Chickpeas and Couscous

Ingredients
1/4 juiced lemon
2 tbsp. olive oil
1 tomato cut into wedges
1 small onion diced

¼ cucumber diced
7 oz. chickpeas
2 tbsp. olives
2 tbsp. fresh basil finely chopped
¼ cup uncooked couscous
Black pepper to taste
Instructions
Cook couscous as per instructions.

Add to mixing bowl then add tomato wedges, onion, cucumber, olives and chickpeas.

Pour over the olive oil and lemon juice and mix until combined.

Place into serving bowl and top with fresh basil.

Chapter 6: Magnificent Mains

Cheesy Baked Spinach

Makes 6

Ingredients

750 grams cooked and finely chopped spinach

200 grams of ricotta cheese

1 cup whole meal breadcrumbs

2 large organic eggs

1/3 cup sliced mushrooms

½ cup green bell peppers

1/2 cup sour cream

½ cup spaghetti sauce

250 grams of sliced mozzarella cheese

1 tsp basil

1/4 cup parmesan

Instructions

Cook and finely chop spinach.

In a large bowl, combine spinach, ricotta cheese, bread crumbs, eggs, mushrooms, and green peppers.

Preheat the oven to 350 degrees F.

Lightly brush a medium sized baking dish with olive oil and spread mixture evenly then spread sour cream on top.

Pour half of the spaghetti sauce across the top and spread with a spatula.

Cover with a layer of mozzarella cheese slices.

Spread remaining spaghetti sauce over cheese slices.

Sprinkle with basil and parmesan cheese.

Bake for 30 minutes.

Cauliflower Italian Style

Serves 4

Ingredients

1 head fresh cauliflower

1 green pepper (de-seeded and sliced)

2 tbsp. olive oil

125 grams of fresh mushrooms

2 tbsp. plain flour

1 cup milk

350 grams of pimento cheese

2 cloves minced garlic

Instructions

Preheat oven to 350 degrees F.

Place cauliflower florets in pan of boiling water and cook for 5 minutes, then drain.

In a skillet add small amount of olive oil and sauté the mushrooms, garlic, and peppers.

Remove skillet and add the flour a little at a time stirring rapidly, slowly add milk while stirring.

Return to the heat and while stirring, cook until mixture thickens.

Place cauliflower in ovenproof baking dish and lay slices of cheese on top then pour the creamed mixture on top of the cheese.

Bake for 20 minutes.

Oven Roasted Chicken Le Mediterranean

Ingredients

300 grams of chicken breast (skinless)
6 large tomatoes (halved)
1 medium onion
1 red bell pepper cut into chunks
¼ cup black olives
4 tbsp. olive oil
1 large courgette (sliced)
250 grams of potatoes (halved)
Salt and pepper (to taste)
1 large tbsp. pesto

Instructions

Preheat oven to 350 degrees F.
Lay all the vegetables in a flat baking dish the sprinkle over the olives.
Make cuts cross ways in the chicken breasts and lay on top of the vegetables.
Mix olive oil and pesto and spoon onto the chicken breasts.
Cover with foil and bake for 30 minutes.
Remove foil and cook for another 10 minutes until chicken is tender.
Serve warm.

South Med Shrimp

Ingredients
500 grams of shrimp fresh or frozen
1 tbsp. chopped finely parsley
1 small chopped onion
1 tbsp. chopped finely oregano
1 bay leaf
2 cloves minced garlic
3 tbsp. olive oil
¼ cup dry white wine
½ tsp salt
3 oz. crumbled Feta cheese
1 ½ tsp cornstarch

ground pepper to taste
1 large can crushed tomatoes

Instructions

Drain tomatoes and keep juice.

Heat skillet over medium heat, add olive oil and sauté the onion, garlic, and spices.

Add crushed tomatoes to skillet with the white wine, salt and pepper cook over high heat for 5 minutes.

Add cornstarch to the tomato juice then add to the skillet and stir, reduce heat and cook until sauce thickens.

Add shrimp and cook until they have turned pink and curled, remove from heat and mix in cheese.

Serve immediately.

Brown Rice with Feta Cheese

Ingredients

1 tsp olive oil
2 medium onions chopped
2 cups brown rice
6 cups vegetable stock
Salt to taste
1 lemon (juice and zest)
4 tbsp. feta cheese

3 spring onions (sliced)
1 tbsp. cilantro (chopped finely)
6 cloves garlic (minced)

Instructions

In a deep pan heat the oil over medium heat and sauté the garlic and onion for 3 minutes.

Add the rice and continue to cook while stirring until rice is coated in oil, about 2 minutes.

Add the vegetable stock while stirring and scraping the sides of the pan until rice starts to cook, season with salt to taste.

Cover and simmer on low heat for 25 minutes then remove from heat and allow to steam for 5 minutes.

Test rice for doneness, if liquid remains or rice is hard return to the heat for a few minutes.

Once cooked, add the feta cheese, spring onions, and cilantro, gently stir until combined.

Serve immediately.

Minestrone Stew

Serves 8

Ingredients

1 can drained kidney beans
2 cloves garlic chopped
Salt to taste
¼ tsp pepper
2 tbsp. olive oil
¼ cup parsley (chopped)
½ cup tomato juice (unsweetened)
1/3 cup whole wheat pasta
2 ½ cups water
1 small zucchini (chopped or sliced)
1 16 oz. can tomatoes
2 large celery stalks finely chopped (include leaves)
2 small diced carrots
1 small minced onion
2 medium diced potatoes
1 cup shredded cabbage
1 cup sliced green beans

Instructions

In a large pan add kidney beans and lightly squash with a fork.

Add garlic, pepper, oil, parsley and salt to taste stir well.

Add water and vegetables, bring to a boil and cook over medium heat while stirring.
Lower the heat, cover, and simmer for 1 hour.
Add pasta, tomato juice, and simmer for 15 minutes.
Salt to taste.

Mediterranean Meatballs

Serves 2
Ingredients
500 grams minced beef
1 tbsp. mint leaves
½ tsp dill dried flakes
½ tsp vinegar
3 cloves garlic (minced)
1 medium onion (finely chopped)
Salt to taste
Pepper to taste
2 slices whole meal bread
1 medium egg (beaten)
Sauce
8 oz. can unsweetened tomato sauce
1 small onion (chopped)
1/3 cup olive oil

1/8 tsp cloves
1/8 tsp nutmeg
1 bay leaf

Instructions

Mix all ingredients and form into small balls.

Flour lightly and lightly fry in a skillet until brown.

Add to sauce and simmer for 20 minutes, add water if needed.

Greek Chicken

Serves 6

Ingredients

1 kg chicken cut into serving sized pieces
3 tbsp. olive oil
5 cloves garlic
2 large onions (chopped)
3 cups Tomatoes (chopped)
¾ cup olives (any type of olives can be used)
Black pepper to taste
Salt to taste
2 tbsp. fresh oregano (or 1 tbsp. dried)
1 cup dry red wine

Instructions

In a skillet add olive oil, place chicken and cook on medium until brown.

Remove chicken and sauté the garlic and onions.

Add tomatoes and olives and cook until the tomatoes are soft, add pepper, oregano wine and chicken.

Cover and simmer for 30 minutes or until tender, taste for salt as the olives can affect the saltiness of the dish.

Serve warm.

Spicy Mediterranean Fillets

Serves 2
Ingredients
2 halibut fillets
1 large tomato (chopped)
¼ cup olives (any variety)
3 tbsp. olive oil
1 tbsp. lemon juice
Salt to taste
Pepper to taste
Parsley 2 tbsp. (chopped finely)
1 tsp cayenne pepper
Instructions

Heat oven to 350 degrees F.

Place fish fillet on a baking tray lined with aluminum foil and season with salt and pepper.

Combine tomato, olives, onion, olive oil, lemon juice in a bowl.

Sprinkle the fillet with cayenne pepper.

Spoon the mixture over the fish and then fold the foil and seal the edges making a large packet.

Bake on baking tray for 30 to 40 minutes.

When serving sprinkle with fresh parsley.

Mediterranean Spaghetti

4 tbsp. parmesan grated

Black pepper to taste

½ cup parsley chopped

½ cup breadcrumbs

2 cloves garlic crushed

3 tbsp. olive oil

500 grams of whole wheat spaghetti

½ can tuna chunks or flakes

Instructions

Cook spaghetti as per packet instructions until slightly al dente.

In a skillet heat olive oil and add garlic and anchovies, stir while cooking approx. 2 minutes.

Stir in breadcrumbs and remove from heat, add parsley and black pepper.

Toss anchovy sauce with hot pasta and sprinkle with cheese.

Serve warm.

Steamed Mussels

Serves 2

Ingredients

250 grams of mussels (cleaned)
1 tbsp. olive oil
1 clove garlic minced
½ can crushed tomatoes
¼ tsp dried oregano
¼ tsp dried basil
1 pinch red pepper flakes
¼ cup white wine
4 oz. whole wheat linguini pasta

½ lemon for garnish

Instructions

In a large skillet over medium heat sauté garlic and when soft add tomatoes, oregano, pepper flakes and basil lower heat then simmer for 5 minutes.

Cook pasta as per packet instructions or until slightly al dente.

Add mussels and wine to the skillet, cover and turn heat to high and cook for 4 – 5 minutes or until shells are open.

Pour over hot pasta and then sprinkle with parsley and lemon juice.

Chapter 7: Daring Desserts

Grilled Peaches with Mascarpone

Serves 2

Ingredients

1 large peach

120 grams of mascarpone cheese

1 tbsp. crushed nuts

Olive oil

Berries

1 large peach (cut in half with seed removed)

Instructions

Brush bottom of griddle pan with olive oil, brush flat surface of the peach halves.

Grill on one side only, when grill marks appear, transfer to serving plate, top with mascarpone cheese and berries and chopped nuts.

Sushi Dessert

Serves 2

Ingredients

1 large tbsp. pumpkin puree

1 medium orange (cut into 4 wedges)

2 sesame energy bars (orange and honey flavored)
Zest of 1 medium orange
2 tbsp. honey
2 tbsp. Greek yogurt
1 large tbsp. sesame paste (tahini)
Cinnamon to garnish

Instructions

In a food processor place pumpkin puree, yogurt, honey and orange zest, pulse until you have a smooth paste.

Place energy bars between two sheets of parchment paper on a flat surface, roll with rolling pin until it is about 2 mm thick.

Place half of the mixture onto each flat bar with a spoon and smooth out, roll the bars to form a round shape.

Cut into bite sized pieces and serve with orange wedges, honey and cinnamon.

Pudding-Rice with Fruit

Serves 4

Ingredients

½ cup basmati rice

3 tbsp. sugar

¼ cup chopped dates (raisins or currants can be used)

4 cups milk (for extra creaminess half and half can be used)

½ tsp cinnamon

1/8 tsp nutmeg

¼ cup nuts (almonds or walnuts chopped)

1 tbsp. orange zest

Instructions

Wash rice and drain.

In a large saucepan add milk and sugar and heat until milk starts to boil.

Add the rice, fruit and cinnamon and simmer over low heat for about 45 minutes, stir occasional.

Remove from heat, add chopped nuts and orange zest.

Pour into serving bowls and serve immediately.

Panna Delight

Serves 2

Ingredients

105 ml whipping cream
1 ½ tbsp. milk
1 tbsp. sugar
1 tbsp. honey
½ tsp gelatin
1 cup berries (any berries you prefer)

Instructions

Add a quarter of the cream to a small bowl and cover with the gelatin, allow to stand so the gelatin becomes soft.

In a saucepan add the remaining cream, milk, and sugar, slowly heat and bring to a boil while continuously stirring.

Remove from heat and whisk in the cream and gelatin mix until all the gelatin has dissolved.

Pour into 4 small containers and chill for at least 4 hours.

When ready to serve unmold onto serving plates.

Top with the berries and drizzle with the honey.

Italian Stuffed Apples

Serves 4

Ingredients

4 apples

1 tbsp. cinnamon powder

¼ cup (any dried fruit can be used depending on preference)

¼ cup brown sugar

Instructions

Preheat oven to 350 degrees F.

Wash and core the apples ¾ of the way so the bottom is still sealed.

Add quarter of the dried fruit to the hole in the apple and top with 1 tsp of the brown sugar then add 1 tsp cinnamon on top of the sugar.

Bake the apples for 1 hour.

Nut Peach Boats

Serves 4

Ingredients

4 peach halves (can use canned)
¼ cup (almonds or any other nuts)
½ ricotta cheese
2 tbsp. honey
¼ tsp cardamom

Instructions

Preheat oven to 400 degrees F.

Cut peaches in half and remove stone (if using fresh), rinse and place facing up onto a small baking sheet.

Mix ricotta cheese with honey and cardamom then spoon ¼ of the mixture into each peach.

Bake for 15 minutes.

Grind almonds in a food processor until fine crumbs have formed.

Gently toast in a pan over medium heat.

Remove peaches from oven and sprinkle with nut mixture.

Lemon Pudding

Serves 4

Ingredients

¾ cup sugar

2 lemons (zested)
2 lemons (juiced)
1 pinch salt
3 egg yolks (lightly beaten)
¼ cup cornstarch
2 tbsp. butter (unsalted at room temp)
2 ½ cups milk
½ cup heavy cream
¼ cup nuts (any variety)

Instructions

Add to a small bowl the sugar and cornstarch and whisk together, add milk and whisk until a smooth paste.

Add the egg yolks and whisk until completely combined.

Pour contents into a small saucepan stir and heat on medium until mixture thickens and sticks to the back of the spoon.

Remove from heat and combine the lemon juice and butter.

Once mixed divide between 4 small dishes.

Let cool and then cover with cling wrap and place in refrigerator to chill about 2 hours.

When ready to serve top with whipped cream and then sprinkle with nut crumbs.

Baklava with Cinnamon

Serves 6

Ingredients

9 sheets filo pastry

8 oz. mixed nuts (chopped finely)

1 tsp cinnamon

8 oz. butter (unsalted)

Syrup

125 ml honey

4 ½ oz. sugar

250 ml water

1 tsp vanilla

Instructions

Preheat oven to 350 degrees F.

Lightly grease a medium baking pan with butter.

Melt butter in a small pan over low heat.

Lay sheets to cover base of baking pan and brush with melted butter.

In a small bowl mix the mixed nuts and cinnamon.

Spread 3 tbsp. over the pastry sheets then cover with pastry sheets, once again brushing each with butter.

Repeat this until you have 2 pastry sheets remaining to cover the last layer of nut mixture.

Using a sharp knife cut a crisscross pattern into top layers of the pastry.

Place into heated oven and cook for about 40 minutes until pastry is puffed and golden on top.

Remove from oven and allow to cool slightly.

Syrup Instructions

In a small pan heat, the sugar, water, vanilla, and honey until the sugar has melted. This will take about 20 minutes stirring continuously to avoid burning.

Pour the syrup into the crisscross pattern you made and let stand to cool.

Cut into small pieces and serve.

Tiramisu

Serves 2

Ingredients

6 medium eggs

8 tbsp. caster sugar

10 tbsp. brandy

Cocoa powder

500 ml black coffee

8 ½ oz. mascarpone cheese

14 oz. sponge fingers

Instructions

Separate eggs and beat the yolks and sugar in a small bowl until thick.

In a separate bowl whisk egg whites until soft peaks form.

Add mascarpone cheese into yolk mixture and gently combine until you have a smooth mixture, now carefully fold in the beaten egg whites.

Mix brandy with the cold coffee into a shallow bowl, dip half of the sponge fingers into the coffee soaking both sides and then place into a dessert glasses or small bowls.

Divide half of the cheese mixture between the two glasses and smooth.

Dip the remaining sponge fingers dip into the coffee and divide between the two glasses.
Top with the remaining cheese mixture.
Chill for about 2 hours in the refrigerator.
When serving cover with cocoa powder.

Luscious Berries and Greek Yogurt

Serves 2
Ingredients
4 oz. Greek yogurt
1 cup Berries any variety
Nuts (any variety chopped finely)
2 tbsp. honey
Instructions
Divide yogurt between two small dishes, drizzle with 1 tbsp. honey and top with berries and chopped nuts.

Chapter 8: Long Term Weight Loss and Heart Smart Achievability

A lot of diets are designed to give a quick fix and rapid weight loss, and although you may be able to achieve your desired weight quickly, there is a good chance it will come back. Also, in following these methods, you will have just been on a diet, and not a change of lifestyle. This is where most people tend to slip back into their old habits and lose all the hard work they have done. This not only means they have to start again, but they become irritable because they have had to start again. Sometimes, they are also the people who say, "this diet doesn't work" so maybe they should switch to the Mediterranean diet and be happy and comfortable.

That being said, as the Mediterranean diet is not a quick fix but a long-term solution to a healthier and happier you. There are several benefits of following the Mediterranean diet. The small amounts of red wine you are allowed to consume have been shown to give health benefits, as with the healthy oils that you will consume on a daily basis. If followed correctly, you can improve the quality of your heart as what you are aiming to achieve is not just weight loss but a long term healthiness. Some other diets can mainly shock your system and can lead to problems, either by losing weight too quick, of depriving your body of the nutrients it needs to function properly.

Other ways to achieve your objectives is to set yourself goals, many of which will happen naturally because of the food that is allowed on a regular basis.

Examples

Goal 1 - change from full-fat milk to skimmed milk, dairy is limited in the Mediterranean diet so that goal is half way complete.

Goal 2 – Reduce dark meat and switch to white meat, this goal is also nearly completed, as dark meat is limited to maybe once or twice per week The diet even goes further and recommends eating fish or shellfish more than poultry.

Goal 3 – Whole wheat bread instead of white bread; this goal is complete as white bread is to be avoided and only whole grains are to be used.

Goal 4 – Water, even though tea and coffee are allowed, it is recommended to set yourself a goal and reduce the amount of these and switch to herbal tea and water.

Goal 5 – Instead of drinking natural juices, try to eat a piece of fruit, this is more beneficial and will also stop you feeling hungry.

Reward Yourself

If you have reached goals that you set yourself, reward yourself, but not with food. Maybe going out with a friend or something you have wanted to do but put off for another day.

Get Help

If you are you are unsure of how to start or plan your meals, a visit to your doctor may help and they could refer you to a dietician. They will be able to advise on how you should manage your weekly menu.

Heart Smart

There are many things you can do to lead to a healthier heart, some of which you have already covered by switching to a healthier lifestyle and the Mediterranean diet. Using healthier oils, as this limits a number of trans fats in your diet, and eating more fish which are full of omega 3. This is good for your heart and your brain. Exercising the recommended 30 minutes per day, as this will strengthen your heart allowing it to pump blood easier around your body. If you have belly fat, this is directly linked to high blood pressure, so once your belly fat is reducing, your blood pressure should lower too.

There are a few more things that you can do which will improve your heart and also your overall fitness. As with all diets, quitting smoking is beneficial, as this has numerous adverse effects on your heart. Keep quiet about this one…a good night of consensual sex is beneficial to your heart!

A visit to your doctor is not just a good reason to get advice, but you should also have a check-up for blood pressure, blood sugar, and your cholesterol levels. You should find the correct levels for your gender and age group, and if you are not currently in range, find out what you need to do to obtain those levels. Having a starting point is also beneficial because if you have a checkup after a month or two, you will be able to see if anything has changed.

A healthy dose of dark chocolate every now and again can help your heart, as it contains heart-healthy flavonoids which help with inflammation reduction. Try to reduce stress levels, or maybe take a different route home to avoid traffic. If you visit or work in an office block that has an elevator, try taking the stairs instead, because this can be used as one of your exercise quotients or even additional exercise. Switching from your morning and afternoon coffee to a cup of green or black tea, as these have been linked to reducing angina and heart attacks.

If you feel agitated or angry for any reason, instead of letting it build up, go for a long walk. This can lower your stress and lead to your blood pressure dropping, and it is also recommended to walk for at least thirty minutes daily. This can be achieved by parking on the far side of the parking lot if you drive, or even walking to work if you live close. If you travel by bus, just getting off one or two stops earlier can help.

One of the main ways to look after your heart is to keep a positive outlook on life. A 'sunny' outlook is good for your mood and blood pressure, although life may get you down, the newfound health and happiness following the Mediterranean lifestyle will be good for you now, and for many years to come.

Conclusion

I would like to thank you for buying this book and I really hope the information which it contains can be of a great benefit to you. As I have continually mentioned, the Mediterranean diet is not just about the food, it will lead you into a better lifestyle. One where you will feel much better about yourself and feeling much better inside.

It is not the end of the road, just the beginning, actually. Also, with the recipes that are included, you will find new ways of either adapting these or finding new ones…or maybe creating your own. I have given all of my insight to what some people are calling, "The healthiest diet in the world." I would actually stand and say, "I do not really call it a diet" as it is a normal way of life and a normal way of eating. Even if some may argue against it, I am sure there are many people in the Mediterranean who live this life every day, and have a different point of view. Not only do they have a different point of view, they can prove that it works by still being active at a ripe old age to prove it!

Part 2

Introduction

The Mediterranean diet plan is a combination of the traditional cooking styles of the countries surrounding the Mediterranean Sea -- from Spain to the Middle East. An increasing number of researchers continue to demonstrate that eating a diet rich in plant foods and "good" fats protects against cardiovascular disease, metabolic syndrome, cancer, obesity, type 2 diabetes, dementia, and Alzheimer's disease.

How to Follow a Mediterranean-Style Diet

☐ Eat mostly plant foods like fresh fruits and vegetables.
☐ Choose whole grains instead of refined grains. For example, eat brown rice instead of white rice.
☐ Make legumes, fish, poultry, and nuts your primary sources of protein.

- ☐ Replace butter with olive oil, especially when cooking.
- ☐ Use herbs and spices to flavor foods instead of salt.
- ☐ Limit servings of red meat to 1-2 times per month.
- ☐ Limit servings of cheese and milk to 2-3 times per week.
- ☐ Drink red wine (optional).

What Foods Should I Choose?

The Mediterranean diet includes...

- ☐ Fresh fruits like apples, strawberries, apricots, peaches, and kiwis.
- ☐ Vegetables like zucchini, eggplants, spinach, peppers, sprouts, broccoli, and cauliflower. Try fresh or frozen options.
- ☐ Whole wheat grain foods like bread, pasta, pita, pizza, and brown rice.
- ☐ Have that bread dipped in extra virgin olive oil (EVOO), but not with margarine or butter. Margarine and butter contain too many saturated and/or trans fats to fit into this diet model.

The primary source of fat in the Mediterranean is extra virgin olive oil. It provides monounsaturated fat, which helps lower LDL cholesterol (aka "bad" cholesterol) and contains the highest levels of antioxidants. Research indicates that a diet rich in olive oil could play a role in the prevention of osteoporosis, heart disease, and some types of cancer.

Nuts, such as almonds, walnuts, and pistachios, are high in healthful fats. Fatty fish like mackerel, sardines, tuna, and salmon are rich in omega-3 fatty acids.

The Mediterranean diet includes a moderate amount of red wine. Men can drink 2 glasses per day while women can have 1 glass per day.

Sample Mediterranean Diet Menu:

1) Breakfast: Greek yogurt topped with berries and walnuts, coffee or tea

2) Lunch: Lentil soup with swish chard topped with tzatziki sauce, hummus and whole grain pita bread on the side
3) Snack: Whole grain crackers and cheese
4) Dinner: Roasted cod paired with a wheat berry salad (cooked wheat berries with olive oil vinaigrette, feta, parsley, and tomatoes) and a glass of red wine
5) Dessert: Fresh fruit drizzled with honey.

The Mediterranean diet is rich in alpha-linolenic acid (ALA), which is found in extra-virgin olive oil. The Warwick Medical School involved participants in a study who consumed more EVOO versus sunflower oil. The olive oil totals were much higher for decreased blood pressure. Lowered hypertension is another benefit achieved by consuming olive oil because it helps keep the arteries clear and dilated. It makes the nitric oxide more bio-available. The healthy fats also make you less likely to.

The health of American people is in decline. Despite the high standard of living many of us enjoy, we often unknowingly compromise our health and longevity. The solution, however, is readily found in the food we eat and in simple, nourishing ways we prepare it.

According to the American Heart Association, cardiovascular disease is the number one killer in the United States, claiming nearly a million lives each year. The American Cancer Society asserts that many lives have been lost to cancer by poor nutrition and an unhealthy lifestyle.

The Mediterranean Diet is rich in vegetables, fruit, peas and beans (legumes) and grains. It also contains moderate amounts of chicken and fish. There is little red meat and most fat is unsaturated and comes from olive oil and nuts. Having a small amount of red wine has been shown to increase the health benefits.

In combination with moderate exercise and not smoking, the Mediterranean Diet offers a scientifically researched, affordable, balanced and health-promoting lifestyle choice.

The 30 Delicious, Quick, and Easy, Mediterranean Diet Recipes

Stuffed Tomatoes

Serving size: Yield: 4 servings (serving size: 1/2 tomato with stuffing)

- Tomatoes are sweet, juicy, meaty, and your best source of the antioxidant lycopene, which may help lower your risk of stroke and various cancers. This recipe is simple: just scoop out the pulp and seeds from a half tomato and fill with a delicious stuffing of crumbled goat cheese, kalamata olives, garlic croutons, and some fresh herbs. At 200 calories per tomato, you'll want to make this dish again and again.

Ingredients:
- [ ] large tomatoes
- [ ] 1/2 cup packaged garlic croutons
- [ ] 1/4 cup (1 ounce) crumbled goat cheese
- [ ] 1/4 cup sliced pitted kalamata olives
- [ ] 2 tablespoons reduced-fat vinaigrette or Italian salad dressing
- [ ] 2 tablespoons chopped fresh thyme or basil

Directions:
1. Preheat broiler.
2. Cut tomatoes in half crosswise. Use your finger to push out and discard seeds; use a paring knife to cut out the

pulp, leaving 2 shells. Chop pulp, and transfer to a medium bowl. Place hollowed tomatoes, cut sides down, on a paper towel; drain 5 minutes. Add croutons, goat cheese, olives, dressing, and thyme or basil to pulp; mix well. Mound mixture into hollowed tomatoes.

3. Place tomatoes on a baking sheet or broiler pan. Broil 4-5 inches from heat until hot and cheese melts (about 5 minutes). Serve immediately.

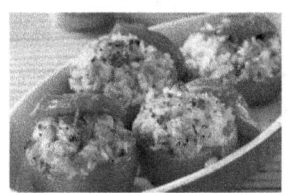

Nutritional Information:
(Calories per serving: 103 Fat per serving: 7g Saturated fat per serving: 2g Monounsaturated fat per serving: 3g Polyunsaturated fat per serving: 0.5g Protein per serving: 3g Carbohydrate per serving: 8g Fiber per serving: 1g

Cholesterol per serving: 6mg Iron per serving: 1mg Sodium per serving: 303mg Calcium per serving: 39m)

Greek-Style Picnic Salad

Serving size: Yield: 10 servings (serving size: 1 cup)

- This recipe is much healthier than your average pasta salad. It packs 4 grams of fiber, less than 300 calories, and delicious, nutrient-filled ingredients like sun-dried tomatoes, spinach, and chickpeas. These ingredients aren't all that common in restaurant-prepared a Greek salad, which makes our take on this recipe even more special. The recipe calls for dried oregano, but if you have fresh sprigs on hand, use a little extra of the fresh herb.

Ingredients:
- [ ] 2 cups uncooked white rice
- [ ] 1 cup boiling water

- [ ] 3/4 cup sun-dried tomatoes, packed without oil
- [ ] 1 1/2 tablespoons olive oil, divided
- [ ] 8 cups bagged prewashed spinach (about 8 ounces)
- [ ] 2 garlic cloves, minced
- [ ] 2 cups (8 ounces) reduced-fat feta cheese, crumbled
- [ ] 1/4 cup chopped pitted kalamata olives
- [ ] 1 teaspoon dried oregano
- [ ] 1/2 teaspoon salt
- [ ] 1/2 teaspoon freshly ground black pepper
- [ ] 1 (15 1/2-ounce) can chickpeas (garbanzo beans), rinsed and drained
- [ ] 3 tablespoons pine nuts, toasted
- [ ] 10 lemon wedges (optional)

Directions:
1. Cook rice according to package directions, omitting salt and fat. Cool to room temperature; set aside.
2. Combine boiling water and sun-dried tomatoes in a bowl; let stand 30

minutes or until soft. Drain and cut into 1-inch pieces.

3. Heat 1 1/2 teaspoons oil in a large skillet over medium-high heat. Add spinach and garlic; sauté 3 minutes or until spinach wilts. Combine rice, tomatoes, spinach mixture, cheese, and next 5 ingredients (through chickpeas). Drizzle with remaining 1 tablespoon oil; toss gently to coat. Sprinkle with nuts; serve with lemon wedges, if desired.

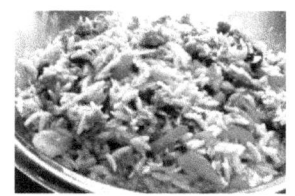

Nutritional Information:

Calories per serving: 288 Calories from fat per serving: 30% Fat per serving: 9.5g Saturated fat per serving: 2.6g Monounsaturated fat per serving: 3.6g Polyunsaturated fat per serving: 1.7g Protein per

Chicken-Garbanzo Salad

Serving size: Yield: 4 servings (serving size: 1 3/4 cups)

- This high-fiber dish, made with chickpeas (garbanzo beans), gets an additional boost of fiber when you scoop it into a whole-wheat pita. The tasty salad is low in saturated fat and high in protein. And, it's simple to make this dish for just one person. (You can even make it and eat it out of the same bowl.) Easy to make and to clean up—that's one of our favorite ways to cook.

Ingredients:
- [ ] 1 (9-ounce) package frozen cooked chopped chicken breast, thawed
- [ ] 1 (15-ounce) can chickpeas (garbanzo beans), rinsed and drained
- [ ] 1 cup chopped seeded cucumber (about 1 small)
- [ ] 1/2 cup chopped green onions (about 4 small)
- [ ] 1/4 cup chopped fresh mint or basil
- [ ] 1/2 cup plain fat-free yogurt
- [ ] 2 garlic cloves, minced

- [ ] 1/4 teaspoon salt
- [ ] 2 cups prepackaged baby spinach leaves
- [ ] 1/3 cup (1.3 ounces) feta cheese with cracked pepper, crumbled
- [ ] 4 lemon wedges

Directions:
1. 18 minutes. Instead of serving this Mediterranean-style salad with pita wedges, make sandwiches. Spoon about 1/2 cup into pita halves lined with extra spinach leaves. With the chicken and the garbanzo beans, you have a protein-packed salad. Yogurt dressing is also a good way to get a boost of calcium and flavor.
2. Combine first 8 ingredients; toss gently. Gently fold in spinach leaves and feta cheese. Serve salad with lemon wedges.

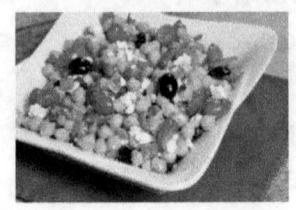

Nutritional Information:
Calories per serving: 258 Calories from fat per serving: 21% Fat per serving: 6g Saturated fat per serving: 2.7g Monounsaturated fat per serving: 1.6g Polyunsaturated fat per serving: 1g Protein per serving: 27.8g Carbohydrate per serving: 22.9g Fiber per serving: 4.9g Cholesterol per serving: 66mg Iron per serving: 2.9mg Sodium per serving: 675mg Calcium per serving: 190mg

Mediterranean Egg Scramble

Servings: 4
Time: 40 Minutes Ingredients: 4 Slices of bread

- Breakfast provides our bodies with the energy it needs to get through the day and helps our brain function. Ever written an exam or given a presentation on an empty stomach? Brain farts galore. I mean, I get it; it's easy to skip breakfast during busy weekday mornings. But making a delicious and nutritious breakfast is easy and takes less than 10 minutes. That's it!

Ingredients:
- 6 Eggs
- ¼ Red bell pepper, diced
- 3 New potatoes, sliced
- 8 Black olives, chopped
- ¼ Cup of fresh ricotta cheese
- ¼ Cup pf fresh parsley
- 5 Teaspoons of butter
- 1 Teaspoon of olive oil

Directions:
1. Begin by heating the olive oil and butter in a pan over medium-high heat.
2. Once the olive oil and butter are simmering, add the sliced potatoes into the pan and sauté for 15 minutes

3. Once potatoes are golden, add the bell pepper and olives. Allow these to cook for about 4 minutes.
4. When this mixture is complete, take a medium bowl and whisk your eggs, ricotta, and parsley together. In your pan, you will want to pour the egg mixture over the potato mixture.
5. Stir the mixture every 30 seconds so that the mixture is firm but not dry. Do this for about 3 minutes. Once mixture is complete, place it over your toasted bread and your meal is complete!

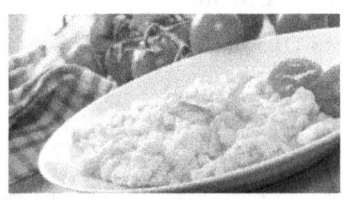

Nutritional Information:
137 calories, 3g fat, 1g sat. Fat, 8mg cholesterol, 19g protein, 7g carbs, 1g fiber, 495mg sodium, 3g sugar

Zucchini and Goat Cheese Frittata

Servings: 4

Time: 50 minutes

Ingredients:
- [ ] 2 Medium zucchinis 8 Eggs
- [ ] 2 Tablespoons milk ¼
- [ ] Teaspoon salt 1/8
- [ ] Teaspoon pepper
- [ ] 1 Tablespoon olive oil
- [ ] 1 Clove garlic, crushed
- [ ] 2 Ounces goat cheese, crumbled

Directions:
1. Begin by pre-heating your oven to 350 degrees Fahrenheit.
2. Next, slice your zucchinis into ¼-inch round slices and set aside.
3. In a large bowl whisk together the eggs, milk, salt, and pepper.
4. Then in an ovenproof skillet heat the olive oil over medium heat, add the garlic and cook for a quick 30 seconds

then add the zucchini slices and cook for 5 minutes.
5. Pour the whisked eggs and milk mixture over the zucchini slices and stir together for 1 minute.
6. Top this with the crumbled goat cheese and transfer to the oven, bake for 10-12 minutes or until the eggs are set.
7. Remove the frittata from the oven and let sit for 3 minutes to cool.
8. Remove from the pan, and slice into four wedges.
9. Serve hot or at room temperature.

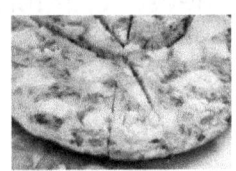

Nutritional information
Per serving Calories: 279 Fat: 24.4g Protein: 7.6g Carbohydrates: 9.7g

Coconut Cookies

Time: 45 minutes
Servings: 4

Ingredients:
- 3 cups shredded coconut
- 4 eggs whites
- 1 teaspoon vanilla extract
- 1 teaspoon lime zest

Directions:
1. Mix the coconut with the egg whites, vanilla and lime zest.
2. Form small balls of this mixture and place them on a baking tray lined with parchment paper.
3. Bake in the preheated oven at 330F for 20 minutes.
4. Serve the cookies chilled and store them in an airtight container

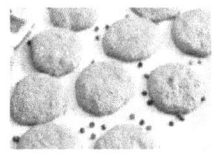

Nutritional information

Per serving Calories: 279 Fat: 24.4g Protein: 7.6g Carbohydrates: 9.7g

Peach Melba

Time: 30 minutes
Servings: 2

Ingredients:
- [ ] 2 peaches, pitted
- [ ] 2 tablespoons honey
- [ ] 2 scoops vanilla ice cream
- [ ] 1 cup fresh raspberries

Directions:
1. Drizzle the peach halves with honey.
2. Heat a grill pan over medium flame and place the peaches on the grill. Cook on each side for 2 minutes or until browned.
3. Serve the grilled peaches with vanilla ice cream and raspberries.

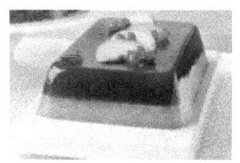

Nutritional information
Per serving Calories: 279 Fat: 8.6g Protein: 4.2g Carbohydrates: 51.0g

Apple Strudel

Time: 1 hour
Servings: 8

Ingredients:
- [ ] 1 package phyllo dough sheets
- [ ] 3 pounds apples, peeled, cored and sliced
- [ ] ¼ cup white sugar
- [ ] 1 teaspoon vanilla extract
- [ ] 1 teaspoon cinnamon powder
- [ ] ¼ teaspoon nutmeg powder
- [ ] ½ teaspoon ground ginger
- [ ] 3 tablespoons olive oil

Directions:
1. Combine the apples, sugar, vanilla and spices in a bowl.
2. Place 2 phyllo dough sheets on a baking tray. Drizzle with oil then spoon part of the filling.
3. Roll tightly then repeat with the remaining dough sheets and apples.
4. Place the strudels in a deep dish baking tray.
5. Bake in the preheated oven at 350F for 40 minutes or until fragrant and golden.
6. Serve the strudel chilled.

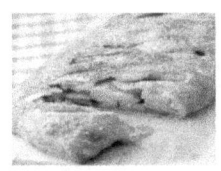

Nutritional information
Per serving Calories: 166 Fat: 5.7g Protein: 0.6g Carbohydrates: 31.1g

Cherry Clafoutis

Time: 45 minutes
Servings: 8

Ingredients:
- 2 cups cherries, pitted
- 1 cup all-purpose flour
- 4 eggs
- 1 ½ cups milk
- 1 pinch salt
- 1 teaspoon vanilla extract
- ¼ cup white sugar

Directions:
1. Place the cherries at the bottom of a 9-inch round baking pan.
2. For the batter, mix the flour, eggs, milk, salt, vanilla and sugar in a blender. Pulse until smooth and creamy then pour the batter over the cherries.
3. Bake in the preheated oven at 350F for 30 minutes.
4. Serve the clafoutis chilled.

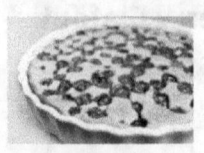

Nutritional information
Per serving Calories: 156 Fat: 3.3g Protein: 5.9g Carbohydrates: 25.6g

Apricot Rosemary Muffins

Time: 1 hour
Servings: 12

Ingredients:
- [ ] 2 eggs
- [ ] 1/3 cup white sugar
- [ ] 1 teaspoon vanilla extract
- [ ] 1 cup buttermilk
- [ ] ¼ cup olive oil
- [ ] 1 ½ cups all-purpose flour
- [ ] ¼ teaspoon salt
- [ ] 1 teaspoon baking powder
- [ ] ¼ teaspoon baking soda
- [ ] 4 apricots, pitted and diced

☐ 1 teaspoon dried rosemary

Directions:

1. Combine the eggs, sugar and vanilla in a bowl and mix until double in volume.
2. Stir in the oil and buttermilk and mix well.
3. Fold in the flour, salt, baking powder and baking soda then add the apricots and rosemary and mix gently.
4. Spoon the batter in a muffin tin lined with muffin papers and bake in the preheated oven at 350F for 20-25 minutes or until the muffins pass the toothpick test.

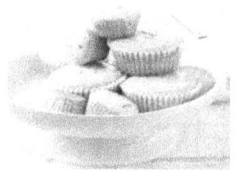

5. Serve the muffins chilled.

Nutritional information

Per serving Calories: 140 Fat: 5.4g Protein: 3.4g Carbohydrates: 20.1g

Minty Fruit Salad

Time: 35 minutes
Servings: 4

Ingredients:
- [ ] 1 cup strawberries, halved
- [ ] 1 cup white grapes, halved
- [ ] 1 mango, peeled and cubed
- [ ] 2 oranges, cut into segments
- [ ] 4 kiwi fruits, peeled and cubed
- [ ] 3 tablespoons honey
- [ ] 2 tablespoons lemon juice
- [ ] 4 mint leaves, chopped

Directions:
1. Combine the strawberries, grapes, mango, oranges and kiwi fruits in a bowl.
2. For the sauce, mix the honey, lemon juice and mint in a bowl.
3. Pour the sauce over the fruits and serve right away.

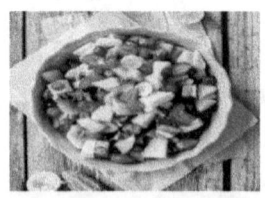

Nutritional information

Per serving Calories: 138 Fat: 0.6g Protein: 1.9g Carbohydrates: 34.4g

Upside Down Apricot Cake

Time: 1 hour
Servings: 8
Ingredients:
- 1 pound apricots, pitted
- 6 eggs
- ½ cup white sugar
- 1 teaspoon vanilla extract
- 1 teaspoon orange zest
- ¼ cup olive oil
- 1 cup all-purpose flour
- ¼ teaspoon baking powder
- 1 pinch salt

Directions:
1. Place the apricots at the bottom of a 9-inch round cake pan lined with baking paper.

2. Mix the eggs, sugar, vanilla and orange zest in a bowl until double in volume and pale.
3. Stir in the oil and mix well then fold in the flour, baking powder and salt.
4. Pour the batter over the apricots and bake in the preheated oven at 350F for 40 minutes.
5. When done, remove from the oven and turn the cake upside down right away.
6. Allow to cool down before serving.

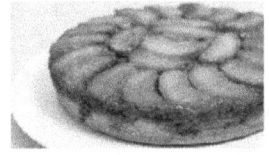

Nutritional information

Per serving Calories: 234 Fat: 10.1g Protein: 6.5g Carbohydrates: 31.1g

Greek Yogurt Pie

Time: 1 hour

Servings: 8

Ingredients:
- 1 package phyllo dough sheets
- 4 cups plain yogurt
- 4 eggs
- ½ cup white sugar
- 1 teaspoon vanilla extract
- 1 teaspoon lemon zest
- 1 teaspoon orange zest

Directions:
1. Mix the yogurt, eggs, sugar, vanilla and citrus zest in a bowl.
2. Layer 2 phyllo sheets in a deep dish baking pan then pour a few tablespoons of yogurt mixture over the dough.
3. Continue layering the phyllo dough and yogurt in the pan.
4. Bake in the preheated oven at 350F for 40 minutes.
5. Allow the pie to cool down before serving.

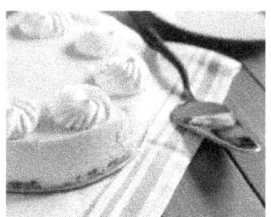

Nutritional information

Per serving Calories: 175 Fat: 3.8g Protein: 9.9g Carbohydrates: 22.7g

Butternut Squash Crumble

Time: 1 hour
Servings: 8

Ingredients:
- [ ] 1 butternut squash, peeled and cubed
- [ ] 1 teaspoon cinnamon powder
- [ ] 2 tablespoons dark brown sugar
- [ ] ¼ cup white sugar
- [ ] 1 teaspoon orange zest
- [ ] 2 tablespoons orange juice
- [ ] 1 cup whole wheat flour
- [ ] ½ cup almond flour
- [ ] ¼ cup butter, melted
- [ ] 1 pinch salt

Directions:

1. Combine the butternut squash, cinnamon, sugars, orange zest and orange juice in a deep dish baking pan.
2. For the topping, combine the flours, butter and salt in a bowl until sandy.
3. Spread the mixture over the butternut squash and bake in the preheated oven at 350F for 45 minutes.
4. Serve the crumble chilled.

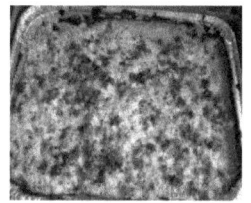

Nutritional information
Per serving Calories: 150 Fat: 5.9g Protein: 1.9g Carbohydrates: 22.9g

Healthy Chocolate Mousse

Time: 20 minutes
Servings: 4

Ingredients:
- [ ] 2 avocados, pitted and peeled
- [ ] 2 tablespoons cocoa powder
- [ ] 3 tablespoons honey
- [ ] ¼ cup coconut cream
- [ ] 1 teaspoon vanilla extract
- [ ] 1 pinch salt

Directions:
1. Combine all the ingredients in a food processor.
2. Pulse until smooth and creamy and serve the mousse right away.

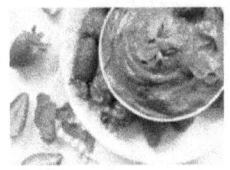

Nutritional information
Per serving Calories: 193 Fat: 13.7g Protein: 1.8g Carbohydrates: 19.7g

Red Wine Poached Pears

Time: 1 hour
Servings: 8
Ingredients:
- [ ] 6 peaches
- [ ] 2 cups red wine
- [ ] 2 cups water
- [ ] ½ cup white sugar
- [ ] 1 star anise
- [ ] 1 cinnamon stick
- [ ] 2 whole cloves
- [ ] 2 cardamom pods
- [ ] 1 orange peel
- [ ] 1 lemon peel

Directions:
1. Combine the wine, water, sugar and spices in a saucepan and bring to a boil.
2. In the meantime, carefully peel the pears and core them. Choose pears that are ripe, but still firm.
3. When the syrup begins boiling, place the pears in the hot oil.
4. Lower the heat and cover with a lid.
5. Cook on low heat for 30 minutes then allow the pears to cool down in the syrup.

6. Remove the pears on serving plates.
7. Continue cooking the wine syrup until it's reduced by half – it will take about 20 minutes.
8. Cool the syrup down in a bowl with iced water and pour it over the pears.
9. Serve right away.

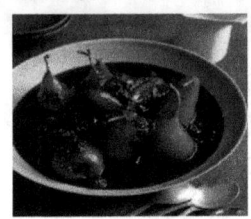

Nutritional information
Per serving Calories: 132 Fat: 0.4g Protein: 0.9g Carbohydrates: 23.0g

Baked Peaches with Amaretti
Time: 35 minutes
Servings: 4
Ingredients:
- 4 peaches
- 8 Amaretti biscuits, crushed
- 2 tablespoons olive oil
- 2 tablespoons light brown sugar

Directions:
1. Cut the peaches in half and remove the pit. Place them with the cut facing up in a baking tray.
2. Top each peach with crushed amaretti then sprinkle with sugar and drizzle with oil.
3. Bake in the preheated oven at 350F for 15 minutes.
4. Serve the peaches warm or chilled.

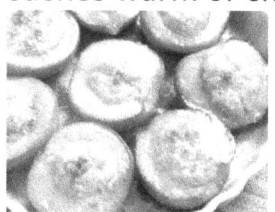

Nutritional information
Per serving Calories: 115 Fat: 7.2g Protein: 0.9g Carbohydrates: 13.8g

Orange Spiced Apricot Compote
Time: 40 minutes
Servings: 6

Ingredients:
- [ ] 1 pound apricots, pitted
- [ ] 2 oz. dried apricots, chopped
- [ ] 2 oranges peels
- [ ] 2 oranges, juiced
- [ ] 1 star anise
- [ ] 1 cinnamon stick
- [ ] 2 cardamom pods
- [ ] 2 cups water
- [ ] ¼ cup white sugar

Directions:
1. Combine all the ingredients in a saucepan and bring to a boil.
2. Cook on low heat for 10 minutes then allow cooling down.
3. Serve the compote completely chilled.

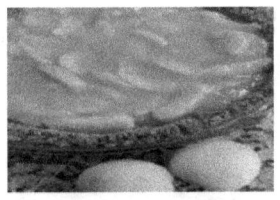

Nutritional information
Per serving Calories: 105 Fat: 0.7g Protein: 1.8g

Coffee Granita

Time: 2 hours
Servings: 6
Ingredients:
- [ ] 3 cups water
- [ ] ¼ cup coffee beans, crushed
- [ ] ¼ cup white sugar
- [ ] 1 teaspoon vanilla extract
- [ ] 1 cinnamon stick

Directions:
1. Combine the water and coffee beans in a saucepan and bring to the boiling point.
2. Remove off heat and allow infusing for 10 minutes then straining through a fine sieve.
3. Place the water back on heat and add the sugar and cinnamon.
4. Cook the syrup for 5 minutes then remove off heat and allow cooling down. Remove and discard the cinnamon.
5. Add the vanilla and pour the syrup into an airtight container.
6. Freeze for at least 1 ½ hours before serving, making sure to stir into the

syrup from time to time to ensure an even, smooth freezing.

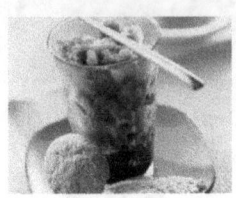

Nutritional information
Per serving Calories: 34 Fat: 0.0g Protein: 0.0g Carbohydrates: 8.7g

Sweet Couscous Salad

Time: 30 minutes
Servings: 4
Ingredients:
- ½ cup couscous
- 1 cup hot water
- ½ cup pineapple juice, hot
- 2 kiwi fruits, peeled and diced
- 1 cup strawberries, halved
- 4 oz. red grapes, halved

- 2 mint leaves, chopped
- 2 tablespoons honey

Directions:

1. Combine the couscous with the water and pineapple juice in a bowl.
2. Cover with a lid and allow to soak up the liquid for 20 minutes.
3. When done, fluff up the couscous with a fork and allow it to cool down.
4. Add the rest of the ingredients and mix well.
5. Serve right away.

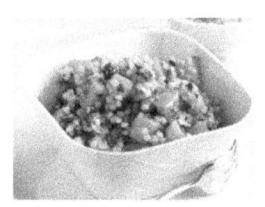

Nutritional information

Per serving Calories: 167 Fat: 0.5g Protein: 3.8g Carbohydrates: 38.2g

Orange Olive Oil Cake

Time: 1 ¾ hours
Servings: 8
Ingredients:
- [ ] 2 oranges
- [ ] ¼ cup olive oil
- [ ] 6 eggs
- [ ] ½ cup white sugar
- [ ] 2 tablespoons dark brown sugar
- [ ] 1 cup almond flour
- [ ] 1 pinch salt
- [ ] ½ teaspoon baking powder

Directions:
1. Place the oranges in a pot and cover them with water. Cook on low heat for 1 hour.
2. When done, allow to cool down then place the oranges in a blender and pulse until smooth. Place aside.
3. Mix the eggs with the sugars in a bowl until double in volume.
4. Stir in the orange mixture then add the oil and mix well.
5. Fold in the almond flour, salt and baking powder then pour the mixture

in a 9-inch round cake pan lined with baking paper.
6. Bake in the preheated oven at 350F for 35 minutes.
7. Allow the cake to cool in the pan before serving.

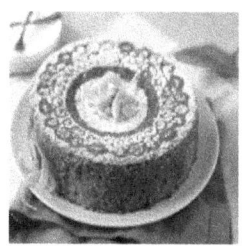

Nutritional information
Per serving Calories: 179 Fat: 9.6g Protein: 4.6g Carbohydrates: 20.5g

Spiced Walnut Cake
Time: 1 hour
Servings: 8

Ingredients:
- ¼ cup hot water
- ½ pound dates, pitted
- 2 cups walnuts, ground
- ½ cup light brown sugar
- 2/3 cup almond flour
- 4 eggs
- 1 teaspoon orange zest
- 1 teaspoon lemon zest
- ½ teaspoon cinnamon powder
- ¼ teaspoon ground ginger
- 1 teaspoon vanilla extract
- 1 pinch salt

Directions:
1. Combine the hot water and dates in a blender and pulse until well mixed and smooth.
2. Add the eggs, vanilla and spices and pulse well.
3. Add the sugar and mix well then fold in the ground walnuts and almond flour, as well as a pinch of salt.
4. Pour the batter in a 8-inch round cake pan lined with baking paper.

5. Bake in the preheated oven at 350F for 35-40 minutes or until it passes the toothpick test.
6. Allow the cake to cool in the pan when done.
7. Slice and serve it fresh or store in an airtight container.

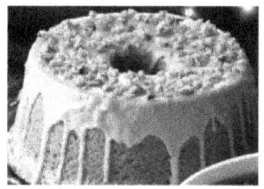

Nutritional information
Per serving Calories: 341 Fat: 20.7g Protein: 11.0g Carbohydrates: 33.7g

Raisins Honey Baked Donuts
Time: 1 ½ hours
Servings: 8
Ingredients:
3 cups all-purpose flour

- ½ teaspoon salt
- 2 eggs
- 1 teaspoon vanilla extract
- 1 teaspoon orange zest
- 1/2 cup milk, lukewarm
- 1 teaspoon instant yeast
- 1/2 cup buttermilk
- 3 tablespoons olive oil
- ½ cup golden raisins
- 3 tablespoons honey

Directions:
- Mix the flour and salt in a bowl.
- In a different bowl, combine the eggs, vanilla, orange zest, milk, yeast, buttermilk, oil and honey and mix well.
- Pour the liquid mixture over the flour and knead for 10 minutes with a mixer.
- Add the raisins and continue kneading for another 10 minutes.
- Allow the dough to rise for 30 minutes in a warm place them transfer it on a floured working surface and roll it into a thin sheet.
- Cut round donuts with a round cookie cutter and place them on baking trays.

☐ Allow to rise for a second time for 30 minutes then bake in the preheated oven at 350F for 12-15 minutes.
☐ Serve the donuts right away.

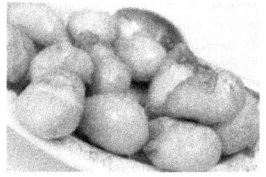

Nutritional information
Per serving Calories: 299 Fat: 7.3g Protein: 7.7g Carbohydrates: 51.3g

Roasted Figs with Rosemary and Yogurt
Time: 25 minutes
Servings: 4
Ingredients:
☐ 1 pound fresh figs, halved
☐ 1 rosemary sprig
☐ ½ cup apple cider
☐ 2 tablespoons olive oil

- [ ] 3 tablespoons honey
- [ ] 1 cup Greek yogurt

Directions:
1. Combine the figs, rosemary, apple cider and oil in a small deep dish baking pan.
2. Cook in the preheated oven at 350F for 10 minutes.
3. When done, remove from the oven and drizzle with honey.
4. Top with yogurt just before serving.

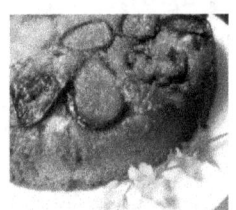

Nutritional information
Per serving Calories: 443 Fat: 9.1g Protein: 8.8g Carbohydrates: 91.1

Ham Spinach Pork Roulade

Time: 2 ½ hours
Servings: 10
Ingredients:
- [ ] 4 pounds pork tenderloin
- [ ] 8 slices ham
- [ ] 2 tablespoons olive oil
- [ ] 4 garlic cloves, chopped
- [ ] 1 shallot, chopped
- [ ] 3 cups baby spinach
- [ ] 2 tablespoons pine nuts
- [ ] 1 tablespoon lemon juice
- [ ] Salt and pepper to taste
- [ ] 1 cup dry white wine

Directions:
1. Heat the oil in a skillet and stir in the garlic and shallot. Cook for a few minutes until softened then add the spinach.
2. Continue cooking on high heat for 10 minutes until the mixture looks softened, but fairly dried out of juices.
3. Remove off heat and stir in the pine nuts, lemon juice, as well as salt and pepper. Allow to cool down.
4. Take the pork meat and place it on a chopping board.

5. Using a sharp knife, begin cutting the meat slowly until you end up with a large sheet of meat that can be rolled later on.
6. Season the meat with salt and pepper and arrange the ham slices on top.
7. Spoon the spinach over the ham then roll the meat tightly to form an even, well wrapped roulade.
8. Seal the roulade with skewers and place in a baking tray.
9. Pour in the wine then cover with aluminum foil.
10. Cook in the preheated oven at 350F for 1 ½ hours then remove the foil and cook for 30 more minutes.
11. Slice the roulade and serve it warm with your favorite side dish.

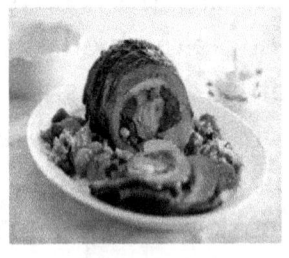

Nutritional information

Per serving Calories: 356 Fat: 12.3g Protein: 51.8g Carbohydrates: 2.7g

Salmon with Salsa Verde

Time: 30 minutes

Servings: 4

Ingredients:

- 4 salmon fillets
- Salt and pepper to taste
- 2 cucumbers, diced
- 2 celery stalks, diced
- 4 mint leaves, chopped
- 4 basil leaves, chopped
- ½ cup chopped parsley
- ½ cup chopped cilantro
- 1 lime, zested and juiced
- Salt and pepper to taste

Directions:

1. Season the fish with salt and pepper.
2. Heat a grill pan over medium flame and place the fish on the grill.

3. Cook on each side for 5 minutes.
4. For the salsa, combine the cucumbers, celery, mint, basil, parsley, cilantro, lime zest and juice in a bowl.
5. Add enough salt and pepper and mix well.

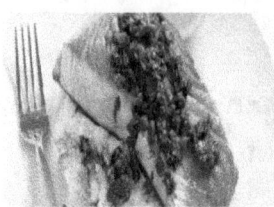

6. Serve the salmon with the green salsa.

Nutritional information
Per serving Calories: 268 Fat: 11.3g Protein: 36.2g Carbohydrates: 7.2g

Baked Sea Bass with Potatoes and Coriander

Time: 1 hour
Servings: 4

Ingredients:
- [ ] 4 sea bass fillets
- [ ] 1 pound new potatoes, washed and rinsed
- [ ] 1 teaspoon coriander seeds
- [ ] 2 garlic cloves, chopped
- [ ] 1 teaspoon Dijon mustard
- [ ] Salt and pepper to taste
- [ ] 2 tablespoons white wine
- [ ] 2 tablespoons olive oil

Directions:
1. Season the fish with salt and pepper.
2. Combine the potatoes, coriander seeds, garlic, mustard, oil, salt and pepper in a deep dish baking pan.
3. Place the fish on top and drizzle with oil.
4. Cover with aluminum foil and cook in the preheated oven at 350F for 30 minutes.
5. Serve right away.

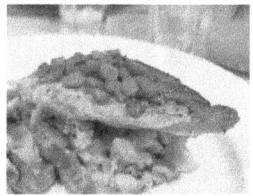

Nutritional information
Per serving Calories: 273 Fat: 9.8g Protein: 25.9g Carbohydrates: 18.6g

Cherry Tomato Caper Chicken

Time: 1 hour
Servings: 4
Ingredients:
- 4 chicken breasts
- 3 tablespoons olive oil
- 4 garlic cloves, chopped
- 2 cups cherry tomatoes, halved
- 1 teaspoon capers, chopped
- ½ cup black olives, pitted and sliced
- 1 thyme sprig

Directions:
1. Heat the oil in a skillet and add the chicken. Cook on high heat for 5 minutes on each side.
2. Add the rest of the ingredients and season with salt and pepper.
3. Cook in the preheated oven at 350F for 35 minutes.

4. Serve the chicken and the sauce warm and fresh.

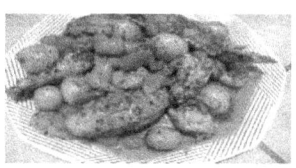

Nutritional information
Per serving Calories: 320 Fat: 19.9g Protein: 30.1g Carbohydrates: 5.6g

Eggplant Ragout Spaghetti
Time: 45 minutes
Servings: 4
Ingredients:
- [ ] 8 oz. spaghetti
- [ ] 3 tablespoons olive oil
- [ ] 1 eggplant, peeled and diced
- [ ] 2 garlic cloves, minced
- [ ] 1 pound ground chicken
- [ ] 1 can diced tomatoes
- [ ] 1 bay leaf
- [ ] 1 thyme sprig

- [ ] Salt and pepper to taste
- [ ] ¼ cup grated Parmesan

Directions:

1. Heat the oil in a skillet and add the eggplant and chicken. Cook for 5 minutes then stir in the garlic, tomatoes, bay leaf and thyme, as well as salt and pepper.
2. Cook for 15 minutes on low heat with a lid on.
3. In the meantime, bring a large pot of salty water to a boil. Add the spaghetti and cook them for 8 minutes until al dente.
4. Drain the spaghetti and mix them with the sauce just before serving, topped with grated cheese.

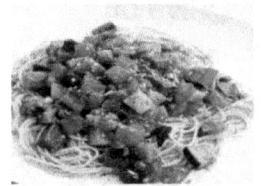

Nutritional information
Per serving Calories: 351 Fat: 14.6g Protein: 28.6g Carbohydrates: 26.3g

Baked Egg in Avocado

Serves: 2

Ingredients:
- [ ] 1 avocado,
- [ ] Halved and pitted
- [ ] 2 small eggs
- [ ] ¼ tsp paprika
- [ ] ½ tsp salt –
- [ ] ½ tsp pepper
- [ ] A bunch of cilantro, chopped

Directions:
- [ ] Preheat oven to 425°F or 220°C.
- [ ] Break an egg into the center of each avocado.
- [ ] Bake for 10 minutes.
- [ ] Sprinkle salt, pepper, and paprika.
- [ ] Top with chopped cilantro.

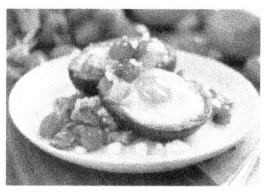

Nutritional Facts
Per Serving: Calories: 222 kcal Total Fat: 18.4g Total Carbs: 10.2g Dietary Fiber: 7.1g Net Carbs: 3.1g - Protein: 7.2g

MEDITERRANEAN DIET

The Mediterranean Diet (or Med Diet) reflects a way of eating that is traditional in the countries that surround the Mediterranean, but you don't need to travel any further than your local supermarket to discover its delicious flavors and fresh foods. It's easy to bring the remarkable health benefits and affordable Mediterranean style of eating to your kitchen cupboards, your refrigerator, your countertops, your stovetop, your oven, and your table every day.

Conclusion

It is my sincere hope that you might have liked all the recipes which have been mentioned in the book and once again thank you for getting this book and experimenting with the recipes.

About The Author

Karen Moran is born with the vision to promote *Mediterranean diet* among the masses. The author has written several research papers on the topic. He has served as an instructor promoting various cultural arts in University of San Francisco. He is currently living with his spouse in Texas.

www.ingramcontent.com/pod-product-compliance
Lightning Source LLC
LaVergne TN
LVHW011950070526
838202LV00054B/4880